Health Benefits of Papaya

For Cooking and Healing

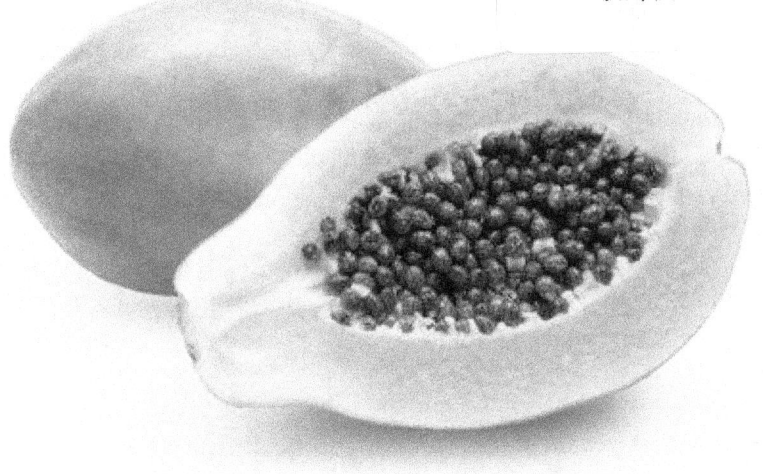

Health Learning Series

M. Usman

Mendon Cottage Books

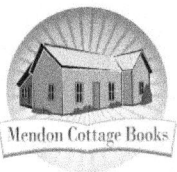

JD-Biz Publishing

Disclaimer

The information is this book is provided for informational purposes only. It is not intended to be used and medical advice or a substitute for proper medical treatment by a qualified health care provider. The information is believed to be accurate as presented based on research by the author.

The contents have not been evaluated by the U.S. Food and Drug Administration or any other Government or Health Organization and the contents in this book are not to be used to treat cure or prevent disease.

The author or publisher is not responsible for the use or safety of any diet, procedure or treatment mentioned in this book. The author or publisher is not responsible for errors or omissions that may exist.

Warning

The Book is for informational purposes only and before taking on any diet, treatment or medical procedure, it is recommended to consult with your primary health care provider.

Our books are available at

1. Amazon.com
2. Barnes and Noble
3. Itunes
4. Kobo
5. Smashwords
6. Google Play Books

Table of Contents

Preface

The deliciously sweet, musky toned and soft papaya is a truly extraordinary fruit which is sometimes even known as the "fruit of angels". This particular fruit was once very exotic and considered a delicacy around the world, but owing to its increasing number of benefits, both health & culinary, the fruit is now being made available all year round in all parts of the globe. The fruit is not only extremely delicious but has several medicinal, nutritional and digestive uses that have sparked the interest of many researches and drug-companies. To find out all about papaya, read on!

Getting Started

Chapter # 1: Intro

Most people hearing the word papaya immediately conjure up images of tropical regions due to its abundant availability & cult status in these places. Papayas are known to have been originated from the Central Americas and are believed to have spread throughout the world from there. Papaya was an important fruit to the Mayans and its tree was called the "Tree of Life". It is believed that when Christopher Columbus discovered the New World, he and his crew became sick from the meager meal of the long sea voyage; the natives took them in, gave them papaya and their sickness went away; this lead to Christopher developing a revered likeness for the fruit.

Papayas are known throughout the English speaking world by different names that are as follows:

i.   North America & Belize: papaya

ii.   United Kingdom: Usually called papaya but also known by the names of pawpaw or papaw.

iii.   Africa: Pawpaw or papaw.

iv.   Australia: pawpaw.

Papayas belong to the genus *Carica* and it is worth mentioning that they are the sole species of this genus. The papaya plant looks similar to a tree, has a single stem that grows 16 – 33 feet tall and has leaves that are arranged in a spiral fashion at the top of the trunk. The lower part of the trunk is scarred and it is here where the fruits are born. The leaves of the plant are quite large, about 60 cm in diameter, and are deeply lobed; the flowers are similar in shape to the species *Plumeria* but are much smaller in size and are more wax-like in texture. These flowers appear on the axils of the leaves and mature into large fruits, about 15-45 cm long and 10-30 cm in diameter. The fruits are pear-shaped or spherical in appearance, can be as long as 20 inches and have an average weight of about one pound. A ripe fruit feels soft to the touch and has an amber to orange color. Their flesh is rich orange in color with either pink or yellow hues; inside the inner cavity, there are many black, round seeds encased in a gelatinous substance. The seeds are peppery in taste, yet edible, but their flavor may prove bitter and unsavory to some.

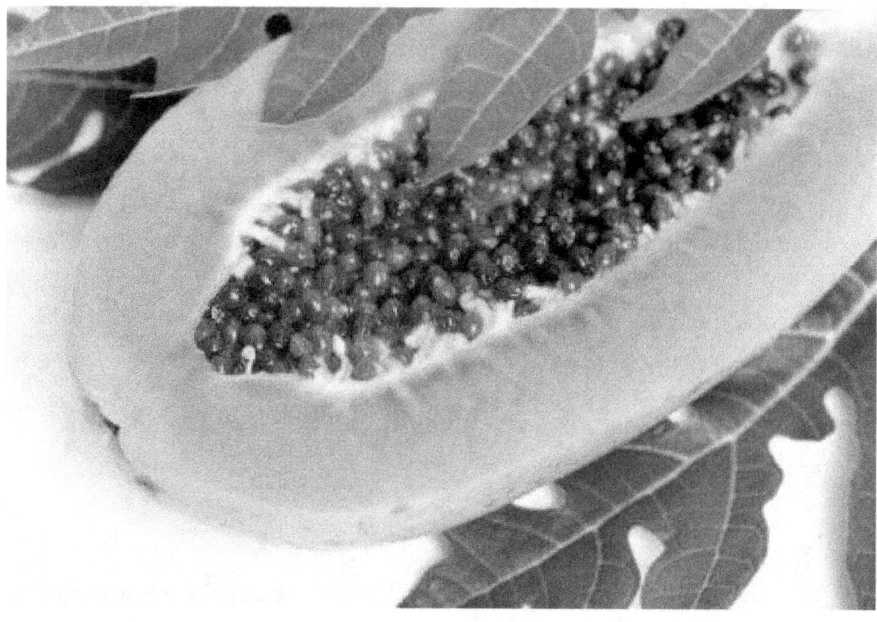

Papaya production throughout the world is highly diversified with the top producers of the fruit spread throughout the world. India is the leading producer with approximately 39% of world share followed by Brazil at 18% and Indonesia at 7%. Other countries with significant produce include Nigeria, Ethiopia, Mexico, Thailand and Guatemala.

Now, coming to the nutritional side of papaya, it should be known that papaya is not only extremely tasty but also very good for health, to be stating moderately! Papaya has a wide range of benefits that encompass the external, as well as, the internal parts of the body.

    i.   **Lowers Cholesterol** – Papaya is abundant in compounds & chemicals that have the ability to lower the buildup of bad cholesterol in arteries that ultimately leads to heart diseases like hypertension & strokes; these compounds include antioxidants and vitamin C.

ii.   **Boosts one's immunity** – The immune system is the body's first line of defense against different varieties of diseases & infections. A single papaya can greatly boost your immunity system with the help of nutrients like Vitamin C.

iii.   **Helps in Weight Loss** – Papaya is very low in calories and therefore can act as a buffer for dieting individuals. Its sweet taste satisfies a person's lust for sugar while keeping the person safe from mass buildup.

iv.   **Helps Diabetics** – Papaya's low sugar content also alleviates insulin levels and sensitivity in diabetics, making it a potential contender for curing diabetes.

v.   **Good for the Eyes** – Papaya has vitamins that can cure age-related diseases like macular degeneration.

vi.   **Arthritis protection** – Arthritis is a very debilitating disease, especially for elders, as it sharply reduces the quality of life. Eating papayas can prove good for the bones due to their anti-inflammatory content. People who consumed foods high in vitamin C, much like papaya had 3 times less chance of getting arthritis.

vii.   **Improved Digestion** – In the 21st century, experimentation with food items is a common fashion and often people perform experiments that turn out to be disastrous for the digestive system! A daily intake of papaya can reduce the chances of a digestive malfunction and improve any bad condition.

viii. **Prevents Cancer** – That's right! This particular benefit will be dealt in detail in a forthcoming chapter, but just as a heads-up, it should be known that papaya can prevent internal parts of the body from damage that later leads to cancer; papaya is most effective against prostate and colorectal cancers.

Chapter # 2: Nutritional Worth

The first and foremost feature of papaya is that it contains no cholesterol; along with zero cholesterol it is very low in calories, i.e. 39 per 100 grams. To be talking statistically, one medium papaya would contain approximately 120 calories, 5 grams of fiber, 18 grams of sugar, 30 grams of carbohydrates and 2 grams of protein; a much more detailed analysis of the nutrients is given below.

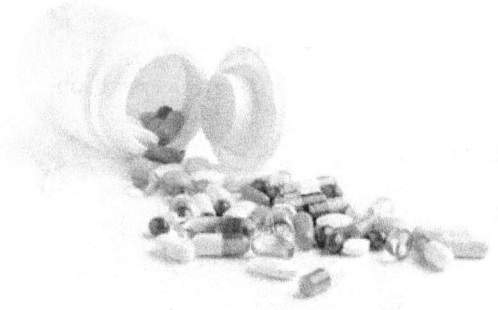

Papaya is rich in nutrients like phytonutrients, vitamins and minerals that have life altering effects on the body, like early prevention of cancer & diseases of similar magnitude. The flesh of papaya is soft & easy-to-digest and is packed with a good amount of dietary fiber, which everyone knows is necessary for a healthy digestive system. In general, papaya has properties that range from anti-parasitic to anti-inflammatory to anti-infectious ones.

Papayas also pack a variety of vitamins in them, namely:

- **Vitamin A** – Papaya is a good source of vitamin A along with many flavonoids like B-carotene, Zeaxanthin, lutein and cryptoxanthin. Vitamin A is a nutrient you must have if one wishes to maintain his/her mucus membranes and keep his/her skin and vision in top-notch condition. The flavonoids are anti-oxidant in nature and act as protective shields against oxidants and free radicals species that play a role in aging and various other diseases.

- **Vitamin C** – Vitamin C is yet another strong natural anti-oxidant that re-strengthens the body's defenses against oxidants and flu-like infections.

- Papaya fruit contains a plethora of vitamin B in it like **Niacin**, **Pyridoxine**, **Riboflavin** and **Folic acid**. These vitamins are extremely essential in the sense that the body is completely dependent on external sources to fulfill these levels.

- Papaya, especially in its fresh form, can prove to be a great source of the minerals potassium and calcium that play important roles in cells, fluids and reactions in the body.

A detailed account of the nutritional wellness of **raw Papaya** is given in the following table. The amount taken is that of a single cup or cubes worth 140 grams.

Calorie Information		
Nutrient	**Amount**	**% DV**
Total Calories	54.6 (229 kJ)	3%
From Carbohydrates	50.1 (210 kJ)	
From Fat	1.6 (6.7 kJ)	
From Proteins	2.9 (12.1 kJ)	
Carbohydrates		
Nutrient	**Amount**	**% DV**
Total Carbohydrates	13.7 g	5%
Dietary Fiber	2.5 g	10%
Starch	~	
Sugar	8.3 g	
Fats & Fatty Acids		
Nutrient	**Amount**	**% DV**

Total Fat	0.2 g	0%
Saturated Fat	0.1 g	0%
Mono-saturated Fat	0.1 g	
Polyunsaturated Fat	0.0 g	
Total Omega-3 Fatty acids	35.0 mg	
Total Omega-6 Fatty acids	8.4 mg	

Proteins

Nutrient	Amount	% DV
Protein	0.9 g	2%

Vitamins

Nutrient	Amount	% DV
Vitamin A	1531 IU	31%
Vitamin C	86.5 mg	144%
Vitamin E	1.0 mg	5%
Vitamin K	3.6 mcg	5%
Thiamin	0.0 mg	3%
Riboflavin	0.0 mg	3%
Niacin	0.5 mg	2%
Vitamin B6	0.0 mg	1%
Folate	53.2 mcg	13%
Vitamin B12	0.0 mg	0%
Pantothenic Acid	0.3 mg	3%
Choline	8.5 mg	
Betaine	~	

Minerals

Nutrient	Amount	% DV
Calcium	33.6 mg	3%
Iron	0.1 mg	1%
Magnesium	14.0 mg	3%
Phosphorus	7.0 mg	1%
Potassium	360 mg	10%
Sodium	4.2 mg	0%
Zinc	0.1 mg	1%

Copper	0.0 mg	1%
Manganese	0.0 mg	1%
Selenium	0.8 mcg	1%

The following is a table stating the nutritional worth of **1 cup of papaya nectar** that is worth 250 grams:

Calorie Information		
Nutrient	**Amount**	**% DV**
Total Calories	143 (599 kJ)	7%
From Carbohydrates	138 (578 kJ)	
From Fat	3.1 (13.0 kJ)	
From Proteins	1.4 (5.9 kJ)	
Carbohydrates		
Nutrient	**Amount**	**% DV**
Total Carbohydrates	36.3 g	12%
Dietary Fiber	1.5 g	6%
Starch	~	
Sugar	34.8 g	
Fats & Fatty Acids		
Nutrient	**Amount**	**% DV**
Total Fat	0.4 g	1%
Saturated Fat	0.1 g	1%
Mono-saturated Fat	0.1 g	
Polyunsaturated Fat	0.1 g	
Total Omega-3 Fatty acids	70.0 mg	
Total Omega-6 Fatty acids	17.5 mg	
Proteins		
Nutrient	**Amount**	**% DV**
Protein	0.4 g	1%
Vitamins		

Nutrient	Amount	% DV
Vitamin A	903 IU	18%
Vitamin C	7.5 mg	13%
Vitamin E	0.6 mg	3%
Vitamin K	2.0 mcg	2%
Thiamin	0.0 mg	1%
Riboflavin	0.0 mg	1%
Niacin	0.4 mg	2%
Vitamin B6	0.0 mg	1%
Folate	5.0 mcg	1%
Vitamin B12	0.0 mg	0%
Pantothenic Acid	0.1 mg	1%
Choline	5.0 mg	
Betaine	~	

Minerals

Nutrient	Amount	% DV
Calcium	25.0 mg	2%
Iron	0.9 mg	5%
Magnesium	7.5 mg	2%
Phosphorus	0.0 mg	0%
Potassium	77.5 mg	2%
Sodium	12.5 mg	1%
Zinc	0.4 mg	3%
Copper	0.0 mg	2%
Manganese	0.0 mg	2%
Selenium	0.7 mcg	1%

Chapter # 3: Selection & Storage

As papaya's popularity grew, so did its cultivation and growth; soon it evolved from being an exotic fruit to a regular food item. It is now available year round in most markets around the world and at an affordable price too; papaya nectar is also available in canned and bottled form. That's not it; some stores even sell papaya in chopped form and in cold cases to preserve its freshness.

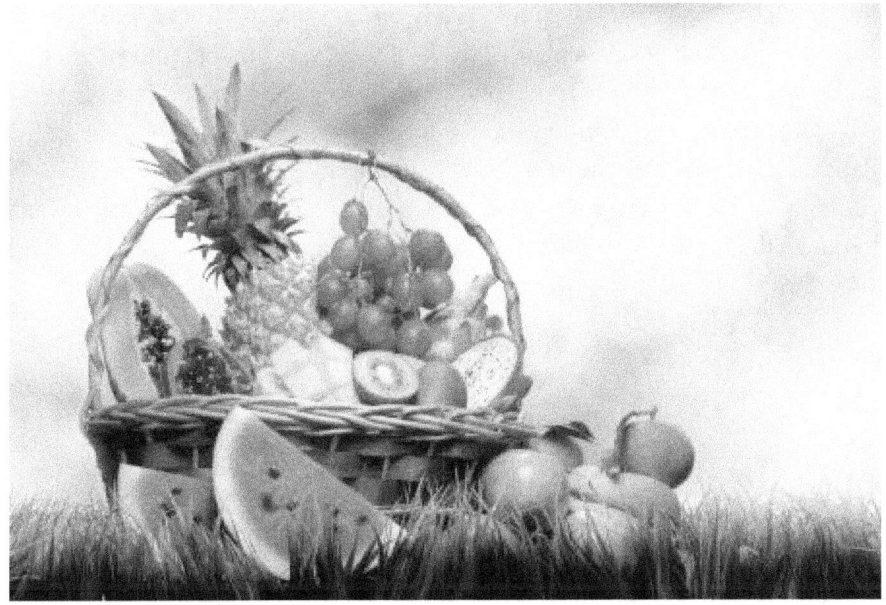

The average papaya is about six inches long and weighs about one pound. However, a larger papaya does not mean a rotten one and papayas can easily weigh as much as 20 pounds. Most papayas are harvested once their skin turns yellow, while organic papayas are left on the tree for ripening; special care must be taken as over-ripe papayas easily fall off which punctures the fruit from one side. When choosing inorganic papayas, choose the ones that are yellow in color and once you take them home, leave them for some time so they can become fully ripe. At reaching ripeness there will be no green spots on the fruit and it will be completely bright yellow in color. A ripe papaya is firm when held and does not yield to gentle pressure; it feels heavy for its size i.e. dense and has a smooth skin free of blemishes. As long as there are no cuts or bruises, a few black spots on the papaya won't affect its health or flavor. Lastly, a ripe fruit also has a sweet aroma. With all that said, green or hard papayas may be purchased if you are planning on cooking them or if you want them for a cold dish like Asian salad.

Papayas will ripen within a few days at normal temperature; if you want them to ripen faster, you can put them in a paper bag. Once ripe, the fruit will turn to mush if not properly stored and therefore should be kept in a refrigerator to halt the ripening process. Place the ripe fruit, in its whole form, in a plastic bag and it should easily last a week. To freeze, peel the papaya, slice it across its length, and scoop the seeds out; cut into smaller pieces and pack these in a rigid container or in a plastic freezer bag. Cover with 30 percent sugar solution and the frozen papaya can last for 10 months. Papaya, in its thawed state will be very soft so if you want to use it in cooking, you might want it in a partially-thawed state; however, if you want to puree, the thawed state won't cause any problems.

Health Benefits

Chapter # 1: Macular Degeneration

Macular degeneration is a term that most people don't even hear about until they are quite old. To start with, macular degeneration, also known as AMD, is an ailment that affects the retina of the eyes; the retina portion of the eye is a layer in the eyeball that has light-sensitive tissues which help in seeing objects. Macular degeneration starts to alter the patient's vision and images that were once quite clear to a person become blurred. Soon, dark spots take over one's vision and become noticeably bigger with the progression of time; most of the sufferers of the disease report straight lines becoming curved and colors becoming much darker. Macular degeneration ultimately leads to partial blindness that only gets worse with time.

Who gets macular degeneration?

- 2% of people with ages above 50

- 8% of people with ages above 65

- 20% of people with ages above 85

So it can be clearly concluded that macular degeneration comes down hard on the elderly and this is exactly where papaya comes in to save the day. An anti-oxidant in papaya named Zeaxanthin has the ability to filter out harmful blue rays that damage the eyes; this leads to better protection of the retina and a decrease in the risk of macular degeneration. Zeaxanthin is actually a carotenoid that can be classified as an anti-oxidant and is found in a variety of fruits & vegetables, most notably papaya. This specific compound has been previously reported to protect against the progression of macular degeneration and has been the subject of many scientific researches since then. Clinical and epidemiological studies have shown that intake of papaya (Zeaxanthin) decreases the exposure of retinal tissues to harmful rays that cause macular degeneration; a much detailed mechanism as to how this happens is still being studied.

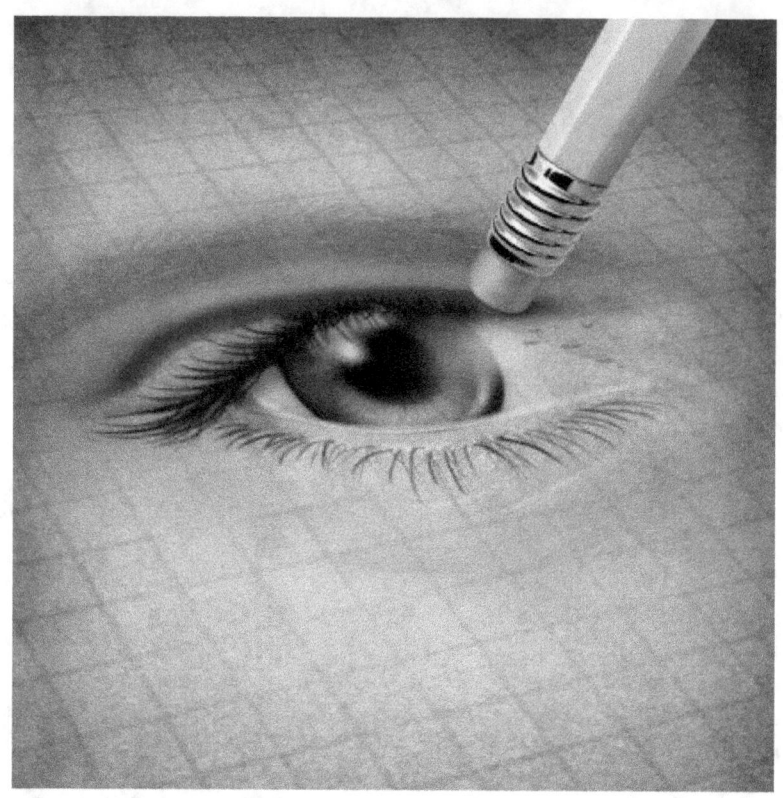

A prospective study was carried out by scientists at Harvard Medical School that aimed to examine the effects of anti-oxidants contained within fruits & vegetables on the development of age-related macular degeneration. The researchers followed the eating pattern of 77,562 women and 40,886 men who were at least 50 years old and had no previous episodes of cancer or macular degeneration. The ages went up to 18 years and 12 years from the baseline for women and men respectively. During follow-up, food intake was assessed with food-frequency questionnaires that were distributed 5 times for women and 3 times for men. Furthermore, during follow-up a total of 464 cases of early ARM and 316 cases of neovascular ARM were diagnosed and it was found that fruit intake was inversely related with the risk of ARM. The data reported showed that participants who consumed 3 or more servings of fruits, like papaya, per day had a lower risk of age related macular degeneration compared to those who consumed less than 1.5 servings a day; the risk reduced by 36% to be exact. It was also found out that individual intake of vitamins and minerals alone did not affect ARM but the intake of fruits had an overall beneficial effect, therefore showing that a combination of vitamins & nutrients was actually the real requirement of the body.

Three servings of fruit may sound like too much, but papaya can help you in reaching this goal quite easily. Add slices of papaya to your cereal, lunch time yogurt & salads and there you have it! Much easier than you thought it would be.

Chapter # 2: Cancer

One of the greatest hazards of the 21st century is a disease known as cancer. Cancer is actually a set of ailments that is mainly highlighted by uncontrolled growth of cells in an organ of the body. There are over 100 different types of cancers, with each one being named after the targeted organ. Cancer affects the body when dysfunctional cells continue to divide uncontrollably, forming lumps of tumors. These tumors eventually grow and interfere with different systems of the body like the digestive, nervous and lymphatic system. Tumors that stay in a single spot aren't as dangerous as:

i. A cancerous cell that moves around the body destroying healthy tissues; this is known as invasion.

ii. A cell that manages to divide and spread throughout the body; this is known as angiogenesis.

A study conducted at the Harvard School of Public Health's Department of Nutrition showed that when diets rich in beta-carotene, a compound found in papaya, is consumed the body is much more protected from the risk of a prostate cancer outbreak. The researchers compared the data of 450 patients who had been diagnosed with prostate cancer from 93-98 with 450 normal individuals, keeping in mind their age, time and year of blood donation. Inverse associations were found between the consumption of beta-carotene foods and prostate cancer growth, showing that fruits like papaya do provide potent protection against the risk of a cancer outbreak.

Colon cancer is another variant whose outbreak and spread is inversely related to the intake of carotenoid rich food items like papaya. A study was carried out at the Department of Gastroenterology at the Japanese Red Cross Hospital in order to find the relation between intake of beta-carotene and the presence of cancerous cells. Serum samples along with lifestyle-altering information were taken from 893 subjects who underwent colorectal endoscopy between the years 01 – 02 and the concentrations of six carotenoids were analyzed in each blood sample. It was found that after all lifestyle-related adjustments had been made; blood samples with the highest levels of beta-carotene had inverse association with cancer development.

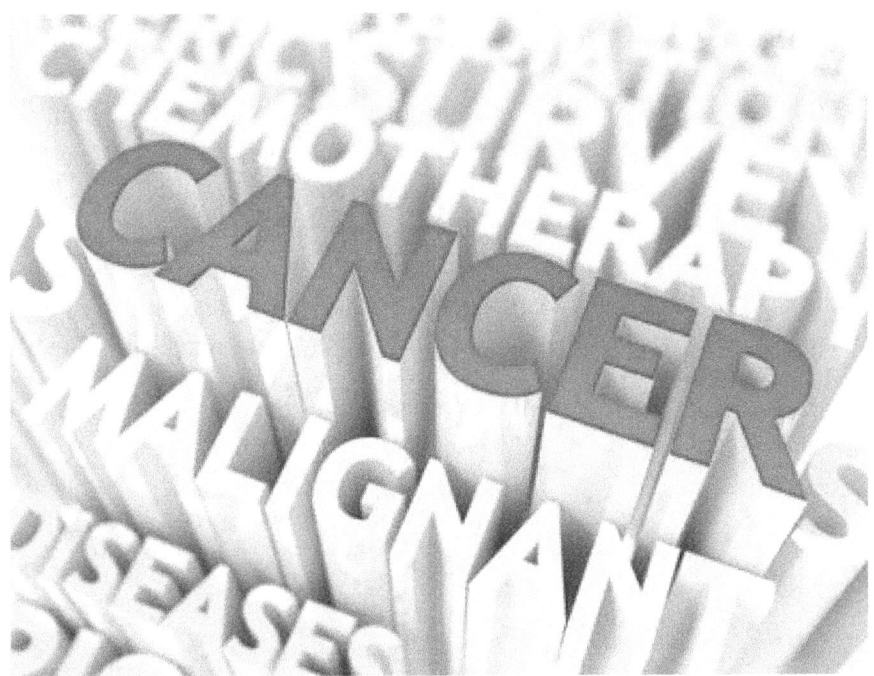

Another research published in the Pacific Journal of Clinical Nutrition showed that the intake of fruits rich in lycopene, like papaya, can greatly reduce a male's risk of developing prostate cancer. In the study, 130 prostate cancer patients along with 274 control individuals who consumed green tea were analyzed for their risk of prostate cancer; it was found that the risk was brought down by 86%. A similar relation was found when lycopene-rich fruits were given to the participants and the risk came down to 82%. Regular consumption of both green tea and papaya had a synergistic effect and offered a much stronger protection against prostate cancer.

A delicious summer snack can be a papaya cut in half sprinkled with lime juice, cottage cheese toppings, and fresh mint leaf along with roasted almonds.

Chapter # 3: Cholesterol

Heart disease is another ailment that is quietly yet swiftly taking over much of the population around the world. Cholesterol, as many might have heard, is one of the major contributors to this disease and therefore, the level of cholesterol in the blood is nowadays used as an indicator for heart disease. As the cholesterol-containing plaque builds up in the narrow arteries and blocks the flow of blood a heart attack is the ultimate result. One way of making sure nothing like that happens to you is by consuming a healthy diet made up of food items like papaya.

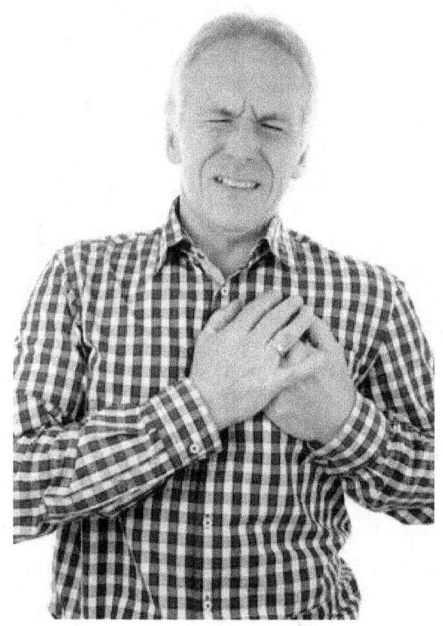

How do papayas work against high cholesterol levels? Papayas are high in vitamin C which is a well-known anti-oxidant. By preventing the oxidation of different compounds, including cholesterol, vitamin C prevents plaque buildup. It should be known that oxidation is one of the steps through which cholesterol deposits in the arteries and blocks the flow of blood. Therefore, it is by this mechanism that papaya helps to increase the flow of blood through the body.

Papayas are also excellent in providing the body with fiber. A diet high in fiber can significantly help lower the levels of bad cholesterol in the body which is directly attributed to causing heart attack and stroke. Furthermore, papaya contains B-vitamins, like Folic acid, which is indirectly linked to preventing cardiovascular damage. It does so by breaking down and removing any circulating toxins, like homocysteine, from the blood which can damage the lining of blood vessels and contribute to increasing the risk of heart disease.

Chapter # 4: Skin Health

As stated in the previous section, papaya's health benefits are not limited to the internal workings of the body, but it works on the outside as well. Papaya is particularly healthy for the skin and this property has been in use by the locals for hundreds of years. Recently, researchers have found that proteolytic compounds, papain and chymopapain are responsible for the benefits provided by papaya to the skin Ointments containing papain are now being used to treat bedsores and ulcers.

The following is a list of comprehensive benefits to the skin offered by papaya:

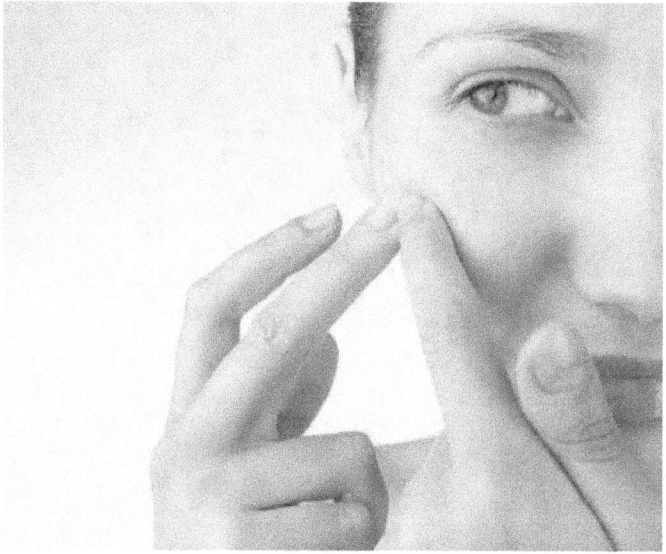

i.   Being an excellent source of the enzyme papain and vitamin A, papaya helps the body get rid of dead skin cells by breaking down inactive proteins in the body.

ii. Papaya also ensures that the skin remains hydrated with its low quality of sodium which means little water is retained after consumption of papaya.

iii. Papaya can help reduce unwanted pimples and blemishes on one's face.

iv. Consumption as well as direct application of papaya will help you achieve supple, smooth and soft skin.

v. Papaya provides long lasting glow to the skin which comes from the inside.

vi. Papaya's paste can be used to treat sores and cracked heels.

vii. Papaya's abundant nutrient store prevents the skin from getting discolored and disfigured.

viii. It acts as the skin's natural exfoliate.

ix. Papaya's peel can be used on the face as well as for whitening one's legs.

x. It can also help in the treatment of ring worms. You just need to rub some slices of the fruit on the patches and see reduced inflammation within some time.

How to use papaya?

To tighten/tone: Puree in a blender or manually mash slices of papaya with several drops of whole milk or whipping cream and apply to your neck and face. Leave it on for 15 minutes and then wash off with water; apply moisturizer afterwards and you should notice tighter skin.

To hydrate/moisturize: Puree in a blender or manually mash papaya along with honey or refrigerated coconut oil and apply it to your face. Leave it on for 15 minutes and finally rinse with cold water. This will have both a moisturizing and toning effect on the skin and will be best for drier and more sensitive skin.

Chapter # 5: Hair Health

Apart from being highly effective for the skin, papaya packs benefits for the hair as well. Papaya contains vitamin Λ which is a nutrient required for the production of sebum, a compound that keeps the hair moisturized. According to hair care professionals, the benefits of papaya for one's hair can be gained by regular consumption of the fruit or by use of hair care products that incorporate papaya extracts.

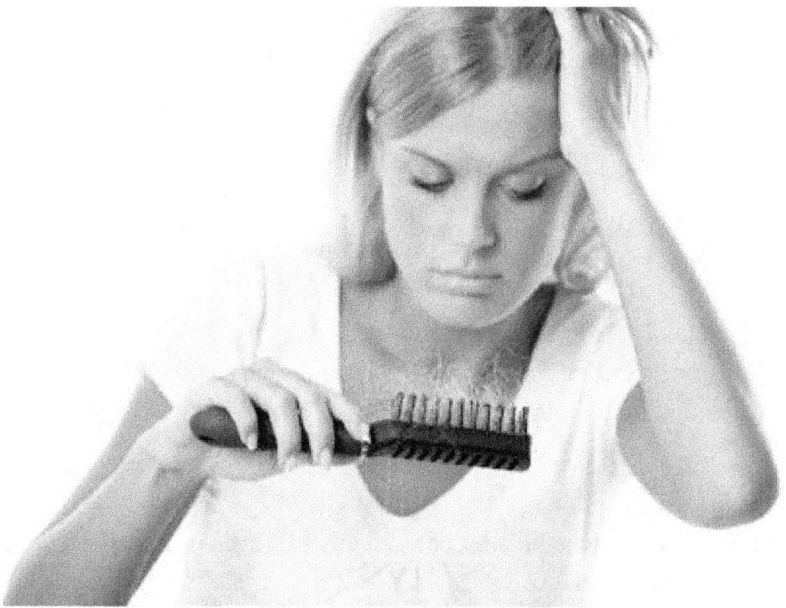

The following are a few benefits of papaya with respect to the scalp:

i.   Papaya can control dandruff.

ii.   Papaya's nutrients work together to help prevent balding, thereby helping boost hair growth and strength.

iii.   Papaya can help prevent hair thinning; although no scientific evidence has shown this to work but many people use this therapy on a regular basis to deal with thin hair.

iv.　　Papaya is rich in vitamins, minerals and enzymes that help in removing oil, dirt and chemical buildup from the hair.

v.　　Papaya extracts add shine to dull and lifeless hair; therefore it can be used as a conditioner.

The following papaya hair mask will help your hair achieve shine, strength and thickness.

Ingredients:

- 1 cup diced ripe banana

- 1 cup diced ripe papaya

- 1 tablespoon coconut oil

- 1 tablespoon molasses

- 1 cup yogurt

Directions:

i.　　Blend all the ingredients listed above, thoroughly; make sure that no chunks are left.

ii.　　Apply the mixture to damp hair and cover with a shower or plastic cap.

iii.　　Allow the mixture to stand for half an hour.

iv.　　Wrap a towel around the cap to generate heat and leave it there for another half hour.

v.　　Finally wash your hair in a regular way.

Recipes

Chapter # 1: Papaya Salsa with Grilled Macadamia Crusted Tuna

Makes: 4 tuna steaks

Prep time: 45 minutes

Cooking time: 5 minutes

Ingredients:

- 2 cups diced papaya

- ¼ teaspoon hot chili paste

- ½ diced red onion

- 6 ounces worth tuna steaks

- 1 diced red bell pepper

- ¼ cup olive oil, extra virgin

- ¼ cup chopped cilantro

- 2 tablespoons lime juice

- 1 clove garlic

- ½ cups macadamia nuts

- 3 eggs

- Salt & pepper

Directions:

First, combine the onion, papaya and red pepper in a medium-sized bowl. Add lime juice, garlic, cilantro and hot chili paste to this bowl and toss the contents to combine; refrigerate the bowl until ready to serve. Preheat an outdoor grill on high heat and lightly grate with oil; brush the tuna steaks with oil and season with salt and pepper to taste. Next, whisk the eggs in a bowl and dip the steaks into the egg and run off any excess egg on the steaks. Press in the macadamia nuts. Finally, cook the tuna steaks on the grill, about 2 minutes for each side and serve with papaya salsa stored in the refrigerator.

Chapter # 2: Fresh Papaya Jam

Makes: 4 pint jars

Prep time: 45 minutes

Cooking time: 20 minutes

Ready in: 5 hours 5 minutes

Ingredients:

- 5 cups mashed papaya

- 1 1/3 packages of dry pectin

- ¼ cup orange juice

- 5 cups white sugar

Directions:

Stir the papaya, pectin and orange juice in a large pot over medium heat until the mixture begins to boil. Stir constantly as the mixture heats and once it reaches boiling, stir in the sugar and let the mixture return to boiling. Once the jam has returned to boiling again, start a timer and let it boil for 1 minute. Next, ladle the hot jam into the canning jars and seal the lids. Allow to cool at room temperature and refrigerate jars that don't seal properly.

Chapter # 3: Papaya Stuffed Chicken with Basmati Rice

Makes: 4 servings

Prep time: 30 minutes

Cooking time: 1 hour 20 minutes

Ingredients:

- 4 boneless, skin less chicken breasts
- 1 papaya, seeded, peeled and sliced
- 1 tablespoon margarine
- 1/3 cup melted margarine
- 1 cup orange juice
- 1 pinch ground cinnamon
- ½ teaspoon ground cinnamon
- 1 can crushed pineapple
- 1 tablespoon brown sugar
- 1 cup crushed berry crackers
- 1 teaspoon nutmeg
- 1 pinch cayenne pepper
- 1 cup basmati rice
- 1 ½ cup water

Directions:

Preheat an oven to 175 degrees Celsius and line a baking sheet with aluminum foil. Lay a chicken breast on your work space and use the tip of a paring knife to cut a pocket in the breast through a slit that is 2 inches in the side. Repeat with other chicken breasts and place the papaya slices in each side, sprinkling them with cinnamon to taste. Dip the breasts in margarine followed by cracker crumbs. Heat 1 tablespoon of margarine in a skillet; arrange the breasts in the skillet and cook until they turn golden brown, which would take about 10 minutes per side. Place the cooked chicken into the prepared baking sheet. Now bake the chicken in the oven for 20 minutes and flip each breast. Continue baking until the chicken is no longer pink and the juices run clear; this would take about 20 minutes. If you have a thermometer, it should read at least 165 degrees Fahrenheit when inserted into the center of the chicken. Now bring the rice and water to boiling point in a saucepan and reduce the heat from high to medium once boiling begins. Cover and let the rice simmer until they turn tender; this should take about 20 minutes. While the rice is simmering, melt the remaining, i.e. 1 tablespoon margarine in the skillet that was previously used to cook the chicken; scrap up any brown bits and add the orange juice, brown sugar, nutmeg, pineapple, ½ teaspoon cinnamon, cayenne and salt & pepper to taste. Reduce heat to medium and simmer for about 30 minutes. Once more, reduce the heat to low and continue simmering until the sauce thickens. Let the sauce cool for some time so it is edible and serve the chicken breasts with rice with the pineapple sauce spooned on top of it.

Conclusion

This book would have definitely shown you that papaya is the "fruit of angels" and truly deserves that title. The fruit is packed with nutrients and minerals that make it as greatly nutritious as papaya's sweetness; along with being extremely healthy it is greatly enjoyed by almost every fruit lover making it easier for one to reap its health benefits. Papayas are truly nature's blessings and should be utilized as much as possible for a healthy, illuminated and satiated life.

Follow the book wisely and you'll surely benefit from it.

References

http://www.123rf.com/photo_11701835_papaya.html?term=papaya

http://www.123rf.com/photo_19121592_ripe-papaya-with-seeds-and-green-leaf-isolated-on-a-white-background.html?term=papaya

http://www.123rf.com/photo_17966053_basket-of-tropical-fruits-on-green-grass.html?term=fruit%20basket%20papaya

http://www.123rf.com/photo_14837727_vision-loss-ad-losing-eyesight-medical-health-care-concept-with-a-human-sight-organ-being-erased-by-.html?term=macular%20degeneration

http://www.123rf.com/photo_15462859_hair-loss.html?term=hair%20loss

http://www.fotolia.com/id/45417819

http://www.fotolia.com/id/49549245

http://www.fotolia.com/id/41000500

http://www.fotolia.com/id/54507728

Author Bio

Muhammad Usman is a distinguished medical graduate of Allama iqbal medical college (AIMC). He is a professional writer who has been in the field for more than 4 years. During this time he has produced 10,000+ articles, blogs and eBooks on various niches related to diseases, health, fitness, nutrition and well-being. He is a regular contributor to several journals related to medicine and surgery. He is the editor of several journals and newspapers.

Check out some of the other JD-Biz Publishing books

Gardening Series on Amazon

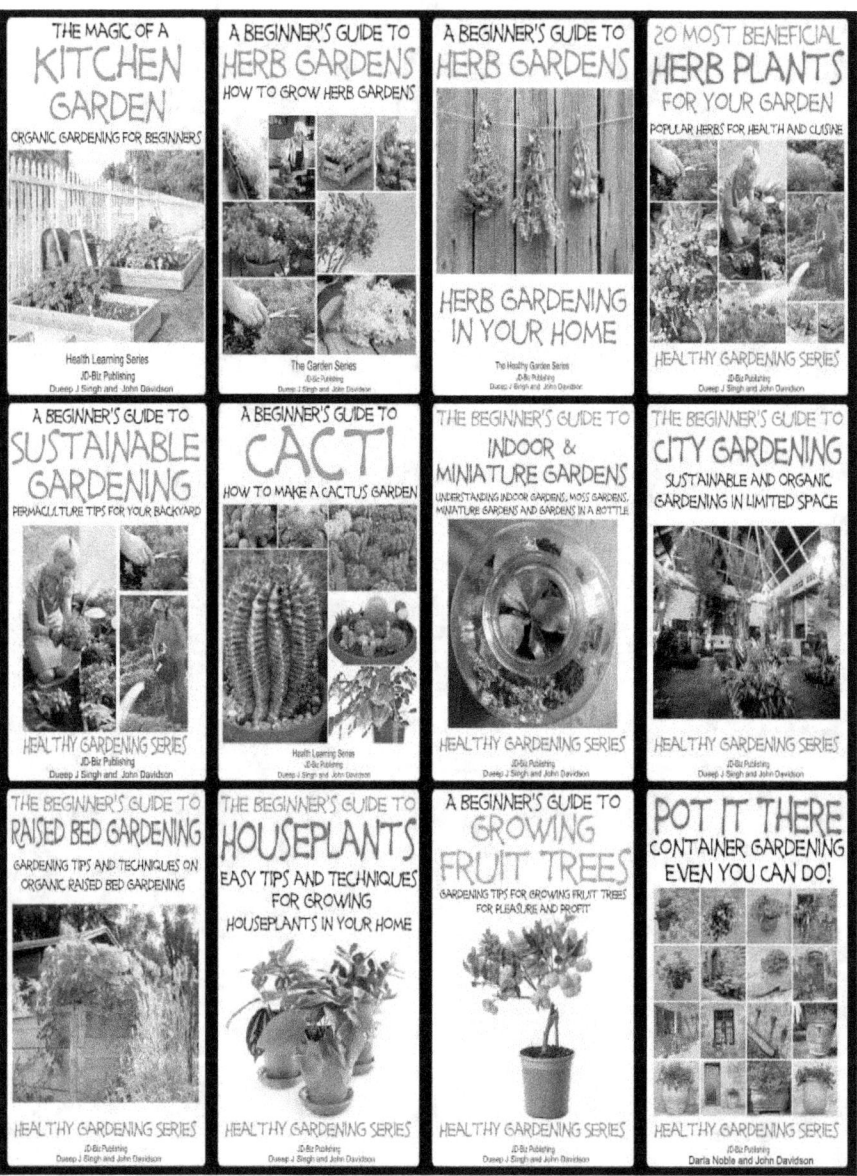

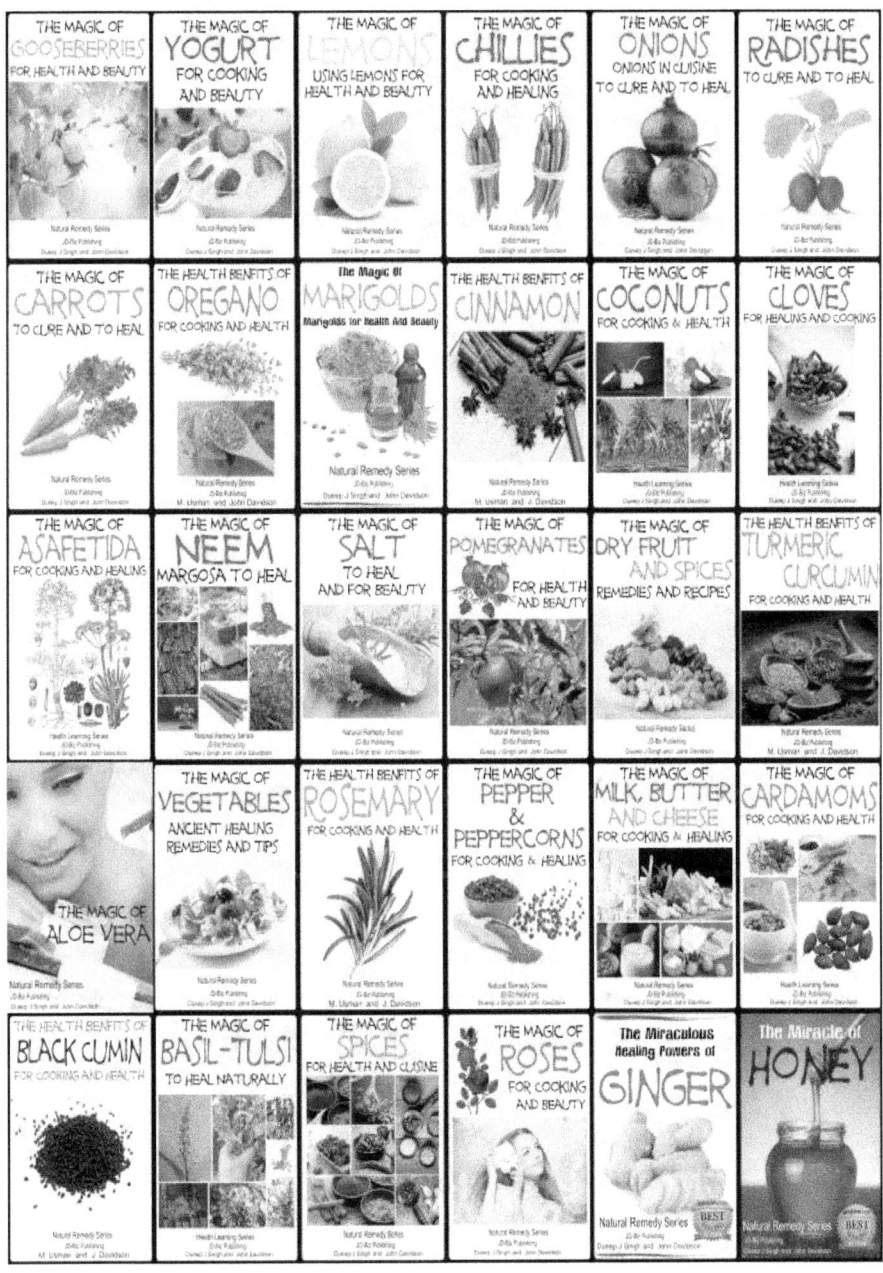

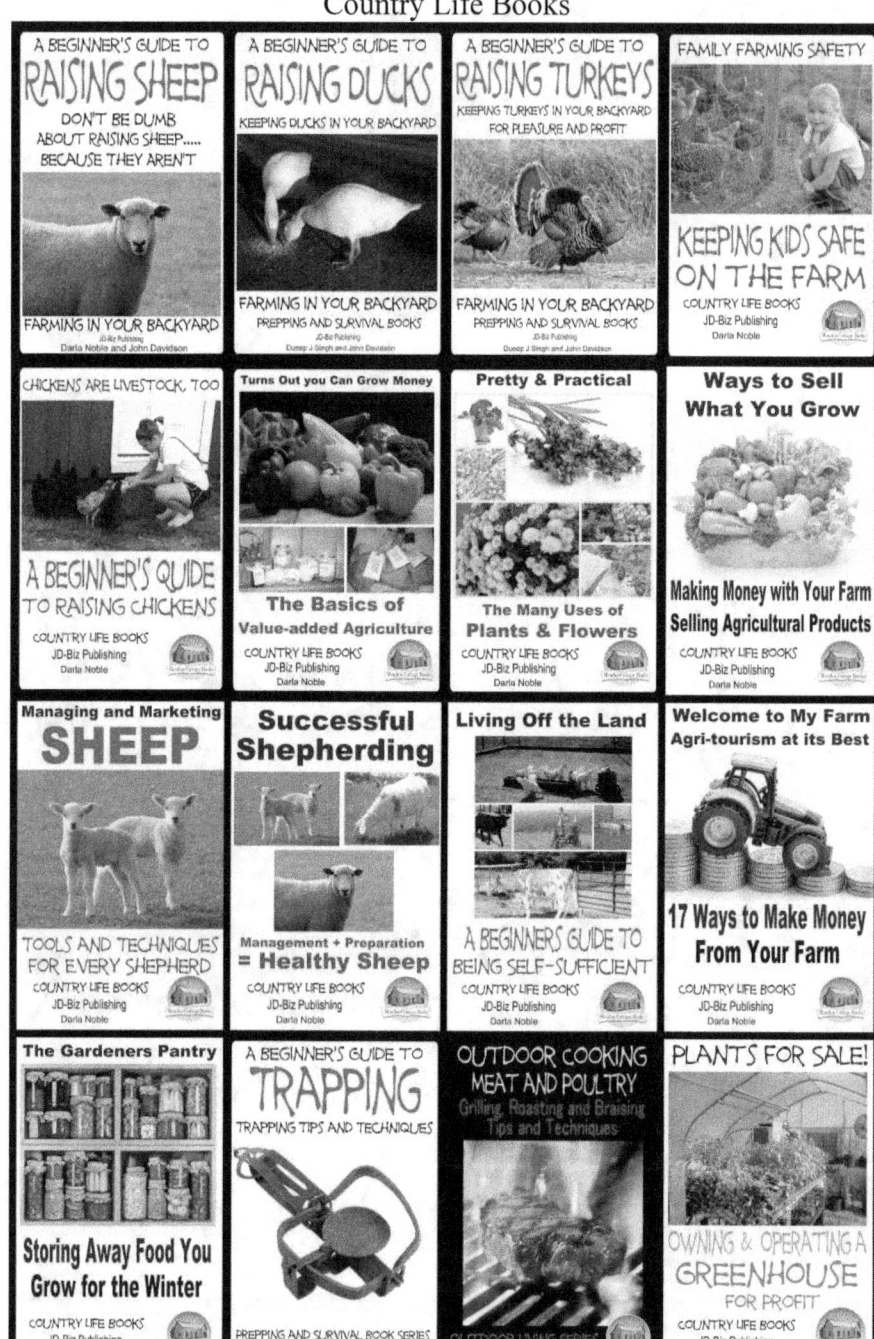

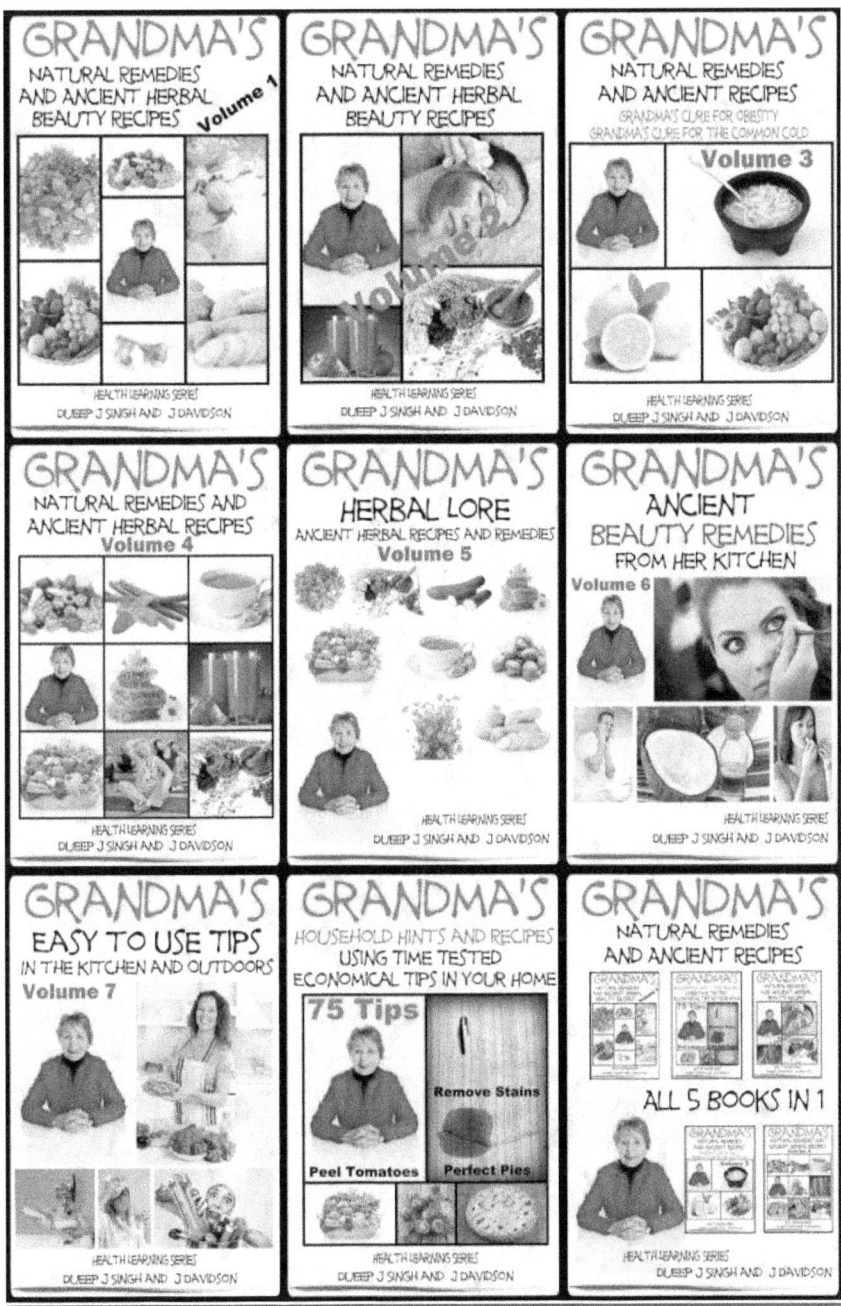

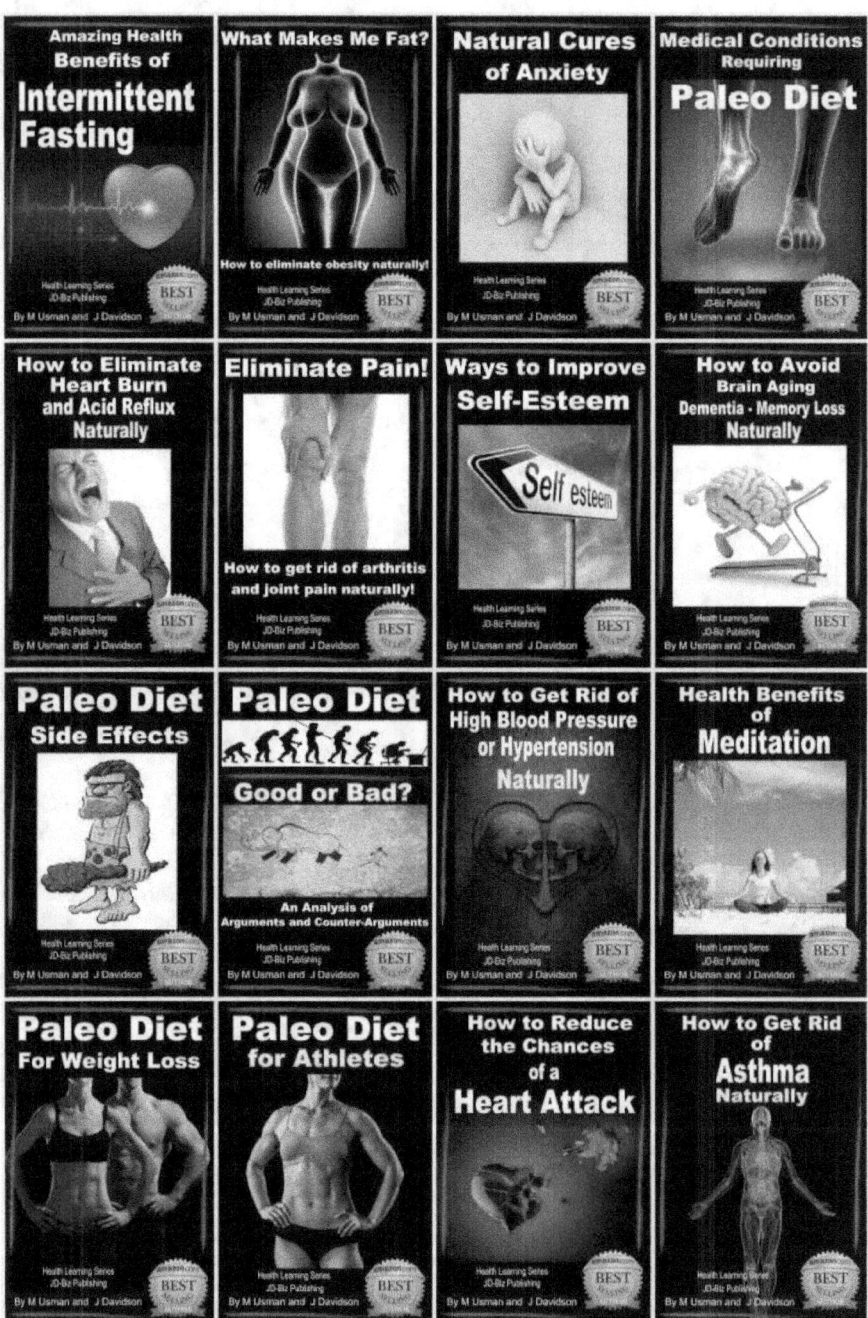

<u>Amazing Animal Book Series</u>

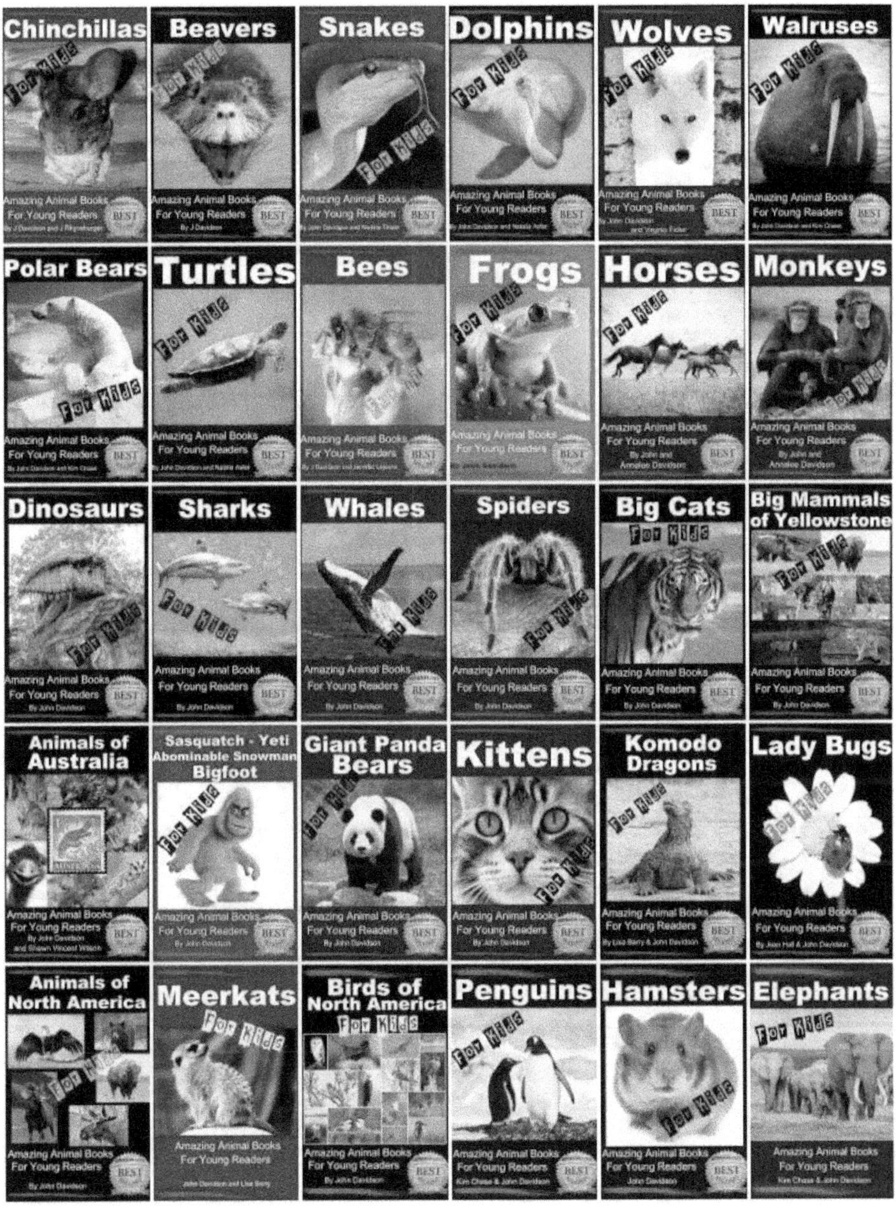

Learn To Draw Series

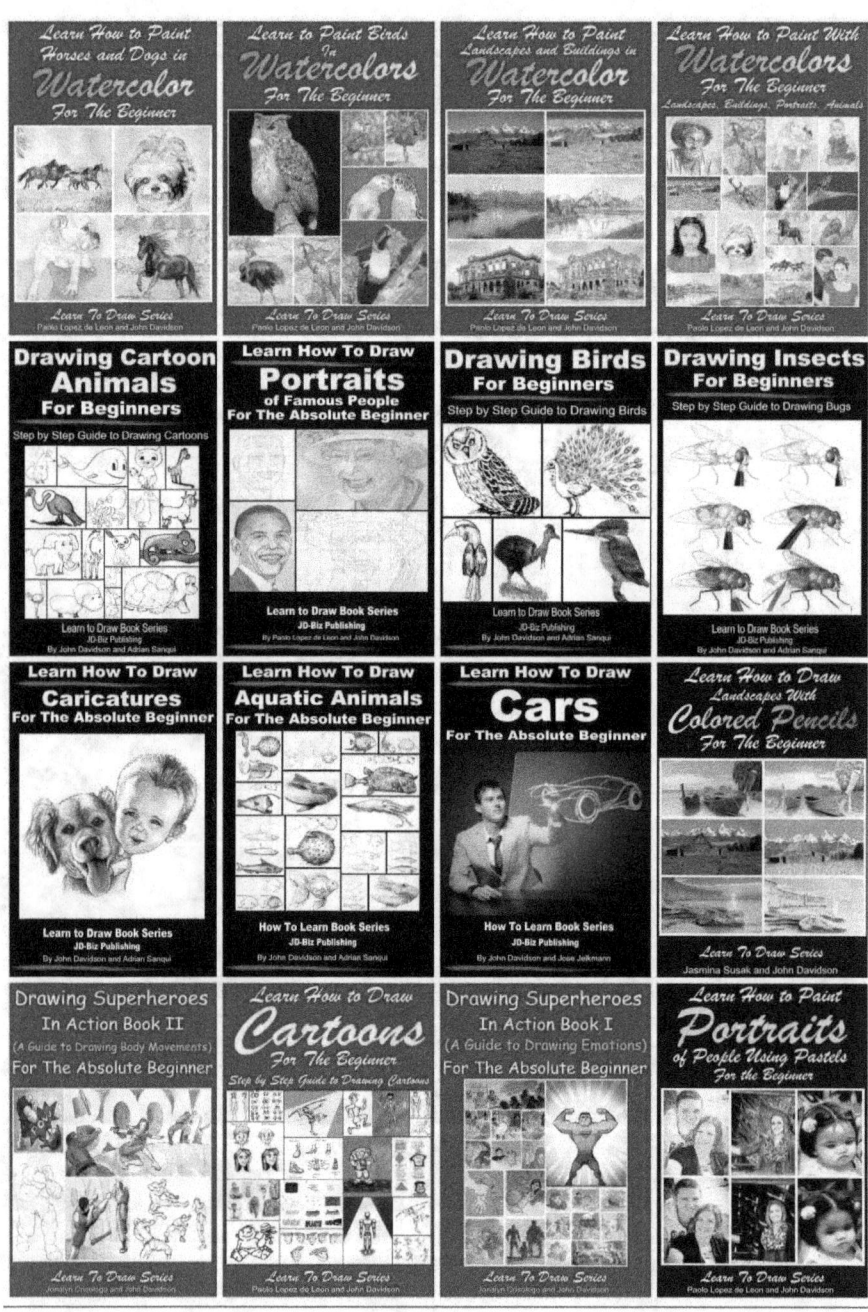

How to Build and Plan Books

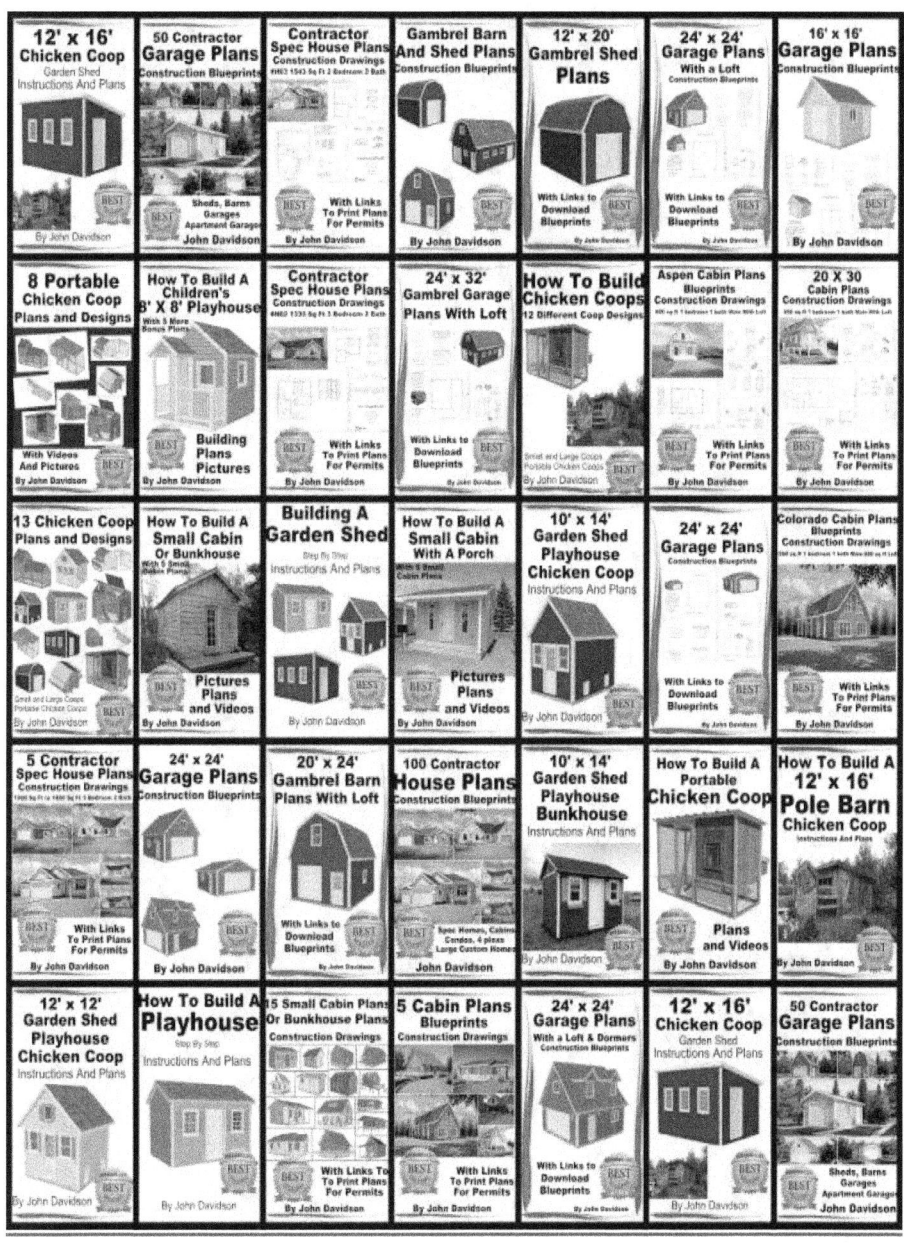

Entrepreneur Book Series

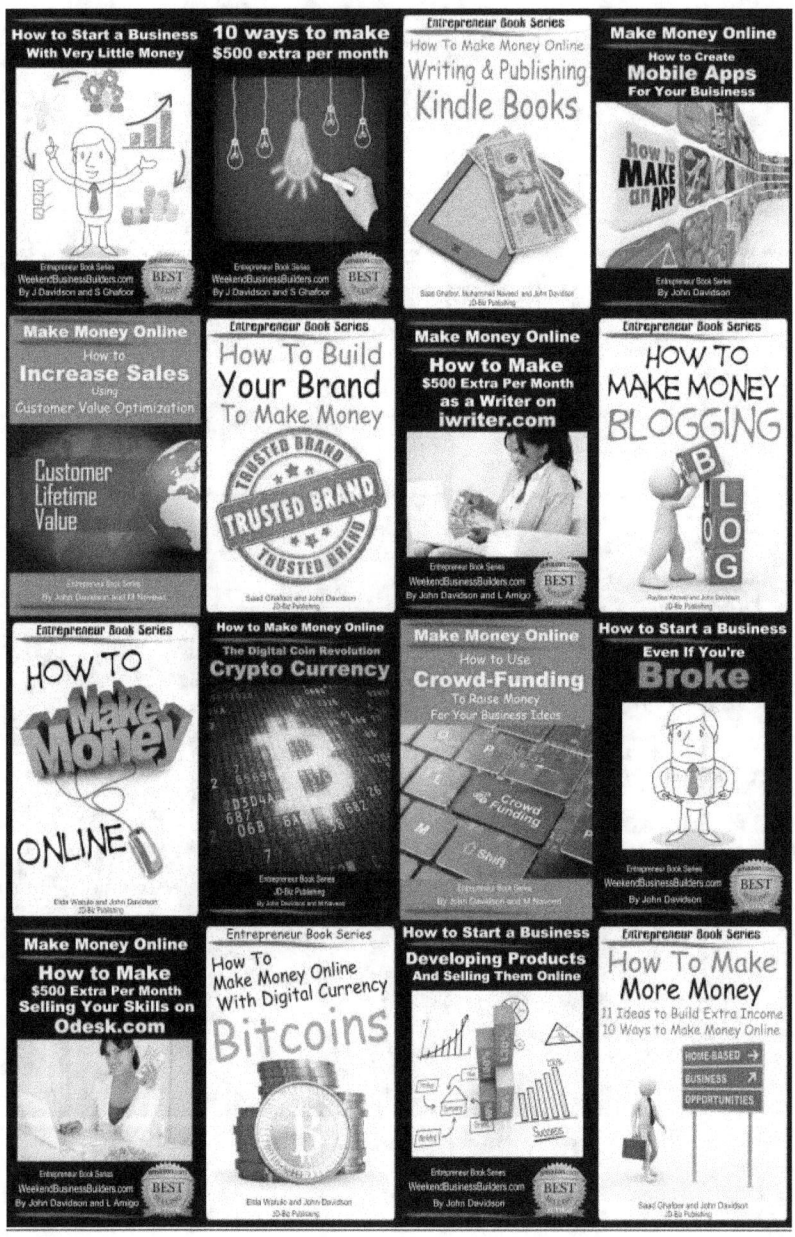

Our books are available at

1. Amazon.com

2. Barnes and Noble

3. Itunes

4. Kobo

5. Smashwords

6. Google Play Books

Publisher

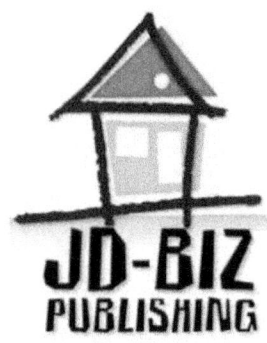

JD-Biz Corp

P O Box 374

Mendon, Utah 84325

http://www.jd-biz.com/

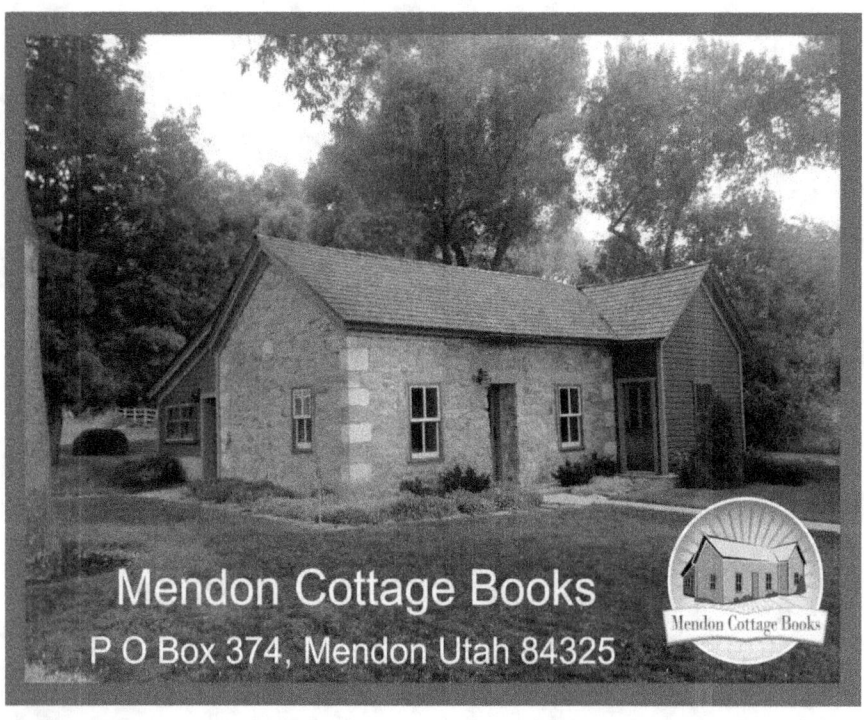

Mendon Cottage Books

P O Box 374, Mendon Utah 84325

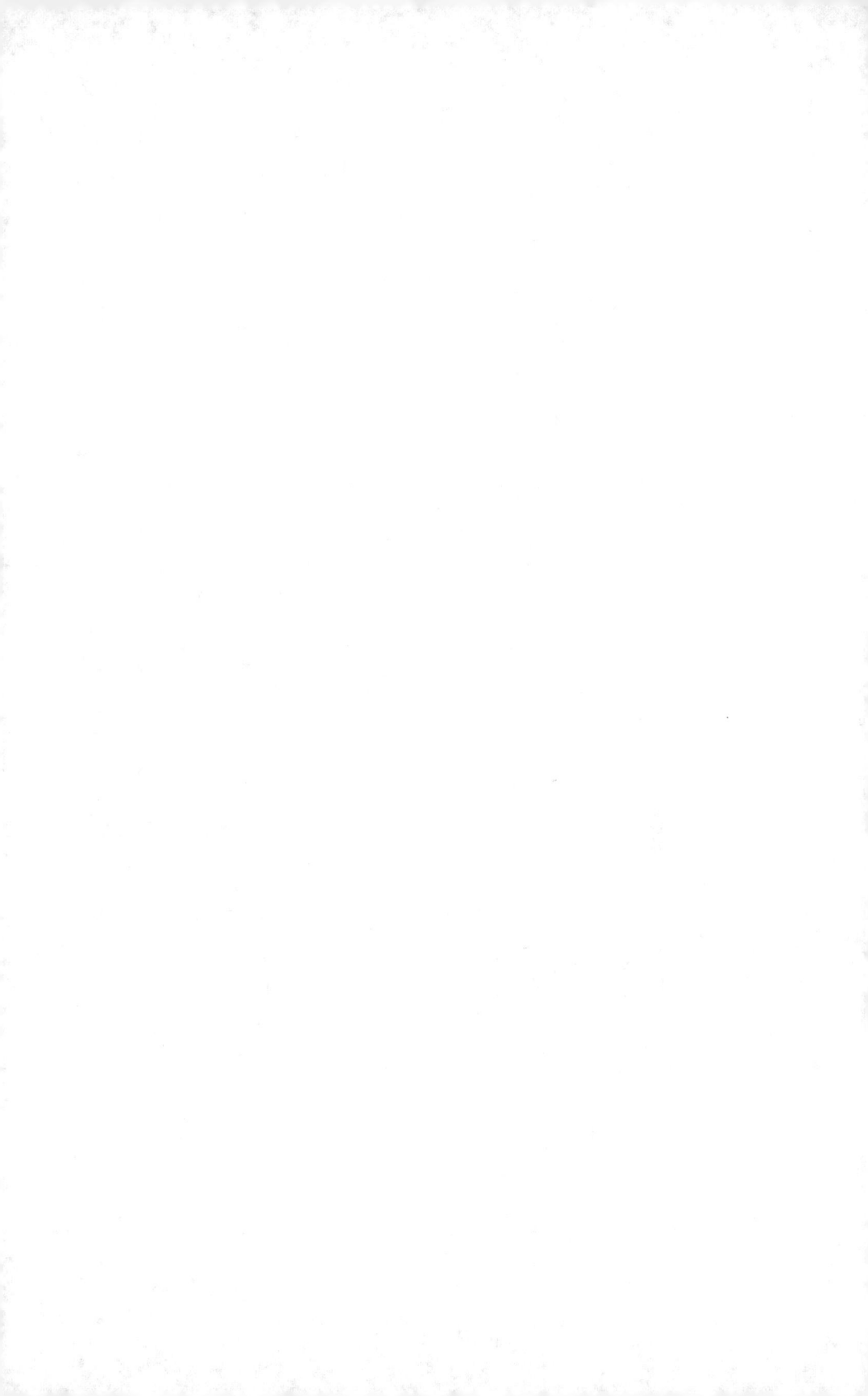

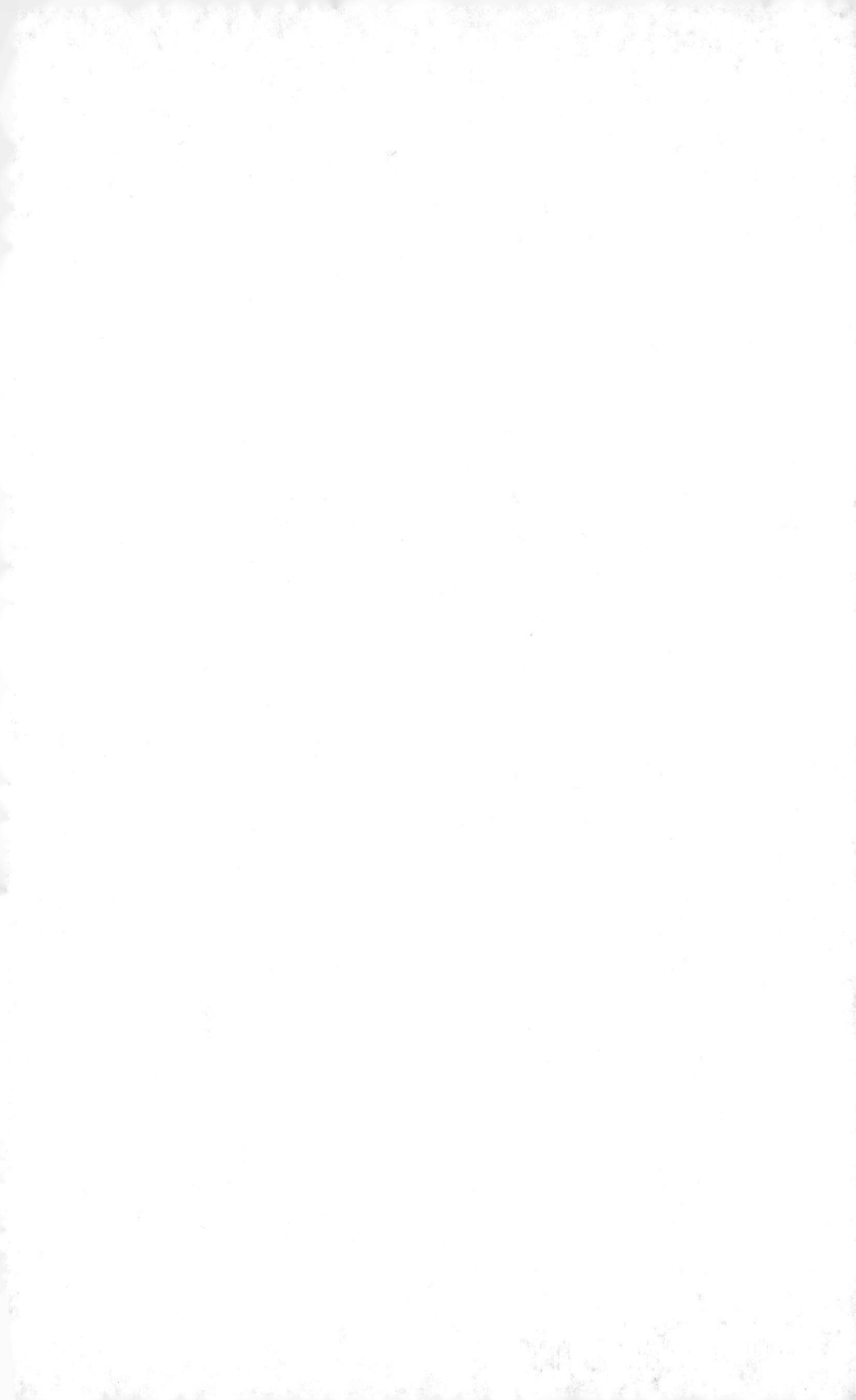